Lust Child

Lust Child

CHILDREN BORN OUT OF LUST AND NOT LOVE

Suave R. Walker

Library of Congress Control Number:		2010908904
ISBN:	Hardcover	978-1-4535-1984-4
	Softcover	978-1-4535-1983-7
	Ebook	978-1-4535-1985-1

To order additional copies of this book, contact:
Xlibris Corporation
1-888-795-4274
www.Xlibris.com
Orders@Xlibris.com
81977

Contents

God does not put on us more than we can bear . . .

This book is dedicated to all those children born into conditions that are totally out of their control. I sincerely apologize for my contribution to bringing another soul into this world in an ungodly manner and not doing things decently and in order. Society would have us believe that it is OK; however, deep within our souls we know that our actions are counterproductive to our religious and moral value systems. Maybe because we have become so undisciplined and have bought into social constructivism. While buying into social constructivism, society as a whole digs itself deeper into the holes of social and spiritual immorality.

Acknowledgments

I would like to thank my Lord and personal savior Jesus Christ, for giving me the courage and the strength to endure, persevere, fight through, make it, and have the courage to write this book without concerns of being judged. He knew that it needed to be told and I thank Him for allowing me to be the vessel that he worked through. Also, many thanks to my parents who supported me in ways that I can only say: thank you for your prayers and for living a righteous life.

My love and gratitude to my dear friends who never judged me and who have always given me their love and support: these individuals have been closer to me than my very own siblings. Gary Sampson, Reginald V. Richardson, Sara Bellamy-Walker, Terri Davis, Tim

Bostic, Lethaniel Griffen, Makeesa Johnson, Ernest Parish, Eddie Deveauex, and Blanton Harris

Special thanks to my son Myles Suave Sherrod Walker for his dedication and commitment to loving me regardless of how I misrepresented myself during my time of indiscretions. He has always displayed respect, concern, and love for me. Very special thanks to the little one. Had he not have been born, this book would have not been written. Through God, I have come to truly love him.

Last but not least, I thank the little one's mother, the person that through it all really displayed character, compassion, and understanding to what I was going through emotionally and was empathetic to me and my situation, while being extremely patient with me in many ways than I care to explain. Nevertheless, again, I am sorry. Without these individuals and their love, support, and prayers, this book and my desire to write it would not have become a reality.

Special Acknowledgments to Brother Hamza Sid Catlett Bey, Dr. Marilyn Volker, Wallace "The Motivator" Durham, Deron Cloud, and Pastor Rennie Blatch. I thank you all for the many times that each of you have blessed me with empowering dialogues and the intellectual, spiritual, professional, and social mentorship that I have received throughout the many years that I have been honored to be acquainted with each of you. My acquaintance with you has been instrumental in my personal growth and development. I cannot express how much I appreciate your contributions to my life. All I can say is thank you!

Foreword

Once in a while a BRAVE man comes along who is willing to address the TABOO sexuality topics in his life, his communities, his world. Then once in a GREAT while, a COURAGEOUS man comes along who is willing to be HONESTLY TRANSPARENT about this taboo topic . . . and to challenge ALL of us to become more honest in OUR lives. This is the CHARACTER of Mr. Suave R. Walker. With great respect, he offers us one of the most difficult, painful, and vulnerable relationship experiences while sharing his private/now public commitment journey. As he details illusions and realities of his life's intimacies involving hurting souls creating an innocent soul, his message is respectfully CLEAR, HONEST, and DIRECT, focusing on his struggles and triumphs regarding RELATIONSHIP COMMITMENT.

With great EMPATHY and HONOR, as the author shares his HONEST SELF KNOWLEDGE and AWARENESS JOURNEY, Lust Child places us in the position of hearing BOTH/ALL souls in continued struggles of commitment, communication, and creation. Mr. Walker not only TALKS his TALK . . . he is willing to WALK HIS TALK by placing himself under the evaluative microscope inviting all of us to assess our relationship commitment and consequences. I applauded Mr. Walker when I first met him as a master's level counseling student at St. Thomas University for his project bridging communication strategies between black men and women and now as he offers ALL communities this written gift of life struggles and life victories. We are blessed to have an author who credits his father (and mother), his faith, and his focus, and I look forward to MORE from Mr. Walker who expects MORE from HIMSELF and more from US.

Dr. Marilyn K. Volker, Sexologist, ABS, AACS
Miami, Florida

Introduction

On Wednesday, December 5, 2007, exactly one year after my divorce and leaving family court, I was in family court again, but this time for child support. How ironic is that? A marriage and family therapist in family court on back-to-back years with family issues that could not be resolved. Unfortunately, I was hit with a brand-new one-thousand-dollar-a-month child-support bill.

Last year my prenuptial agreement saved me, but not this time—I had to pay the little one his in cash and not in time and gifts. Initially, I was a little bitter, but as today passed I got past it. But the nerve of her, there was never anything that I would not do for the little one, so why would she do this to me? I never at anytime breached our agreement that I would basically cover all his expenses. So why do I feel screwed? Oh well, a brother got to do what a brother got to do.

Speaking of doing what I got to do, maybe I will discuss this topic on my radio talk show. I would sure love to hear what my radio family has to say about this Mind-blowing, Thought-provoking, and Eye-opening topic. Or maybe I will write about it.

Lust Child
Children Born Out of Lust and Not Love

There's an old saying . . . . A baby won't keep a man. Many people rationalize that if the couple—or, should I say, the two individuals—conceive a child, it will bring them closer together or even make one of the individuals commit. NOT! Seriously, not necessarily. Children at times are not part of the scenario; it is about sexual gratification and lust by two irresponsible individuals.

Too many individuals have this belief system regardless of the fact that we see, over and over the years, mothers and children abandoned by their father or biological contributors (sperm donors). This pattern of repetition perpetuates the American crisis of single parenting. Most people don't perceive this as a crisis, but they should consider that out of the millions of individuals that live in poverty and suffer from substance abuse and are incarcerated, most come from single parent homes.

I believe you will reconsider your opinion after reading this. According to Oxford's dictionary, crisis is defined as a time of acute danger or a difficult decisive moment. Now that we have a definition of crisis, we can see that it is a time of difficulty.

There are difficulties first within the family structure because there are not enough positive male or father figures within the home or family. There is a time of difficulty when so many homes are headed by women resulting in more young men being raised in a matriarch household. They have no other influence other than grandmother, auntie, and sister, or other female friends and relatives of the family and of course mother. This makes it extremely difficult for the average male to really identify with his MALEHOOD.

These are times of difficulties when out of 100 percent of individuals that are incarcerated, 77 percent come from single-parent households. However, out of the 77 percent, 76 percent are from single-parent households that are headed by females. In my humble opinion, this definitely qualifies as a CRISIS.

Dedication to all those men who struggle with doing the right thing: remember they didn't ask to be here!

Chapter 1

The Breakup

My ex-wife and I were not getting along. We tried counseling, therapy, prayer, and separation, but nothing seemed to work; therefore, we agreed that a divorce was the only option.

I filed for a divorce. This was something that I did not want to experience especially for a second time. Nevertheless, I filed and waited. In the meantime, I continued my studies and stayed focused on being the best father I could be. After all else failed, I was still an excellent father.

During the waiting game, I experienced many emotions, so many that it became so confusing. In fact, I cried because I was confused, because I did not know why I was crying. I was a HOT MESS. No one at work ever knew any of the hardships that I was experiencing because I masked all the pain and torment that I was experiencing. I did not want anyone to know that I was experiencing a divorce and especially those who knew that I had been married before.

One could not imagine the pain alongside the shame a family advocate, and marriage and family therapist has to endure. Especially, when people discover that I could not work out my own marriage. Individuals that are aware that your profession is in the psychology, counseling, or mental health arena tend to take your expertise for granted because they are familiar with you. They tend to not take you seriously.

Therefore, in the dynamic of a marriage, in my case, it was impossible to do. I was never interested in having professional marriage and especially not a therapeutic one. So please do not take for granted that anyone in this profession or any profession dealing with people have perfect or near-perfect relationships. In fact, I am often asked, "Wow, you are a marriage and family therapist and you got divorced, why couldn't you work out your own marriage?" Well, I will never feel guilty for things that other people do; however, I will respond to their question. I normally present this question to them: Are you responsible for your spouse if they are involved with drugs and alcohol? Now this may come off as a bit offensive, but we all know that most people say things without putting much thought into what they are saying.

What I do notice is that when you force people to use their greatest asset, which is their brain, they tend to put a little more thought into the comment that they have just made. And coupled with how defensive your stance was, suddenly you hear this, "Yeah, I really didn't think of it that way."

So as the divorce was being processed, I was trying to adjust to no longer being married and having my wife next to me each night. Now, although marriage with her was a bit challenging, there is that sense of security that both men and women get during a marriage. Nevertheless, I was adjusting, except from time to time when my wife and I would speak on different issues about our marriage. It would just turn to an all-out argument, which would trigger why I was divorcing her in the first place.

I know that breakups are hard, but for god's sake, why do they have to be so ugly? And to think, two people at one point really and truly loved each other and said that they would honor, love one another until death. Well, I guess today we collectively don't really honor our commitments. In fact, we don't honor our commitments, obligations, or contracts. I believe until we collectively, but specifically as men, learn to honor our contract, our lives will not significantly improve.

See, we have to be mentored, taught, and consistently have a committed mind-set to honor our contracts until it becomes second nature. Over the years, we have failed to honor our contracts. We don't honor our contract with our families. We don't honor our contract with our children.

We don't honor our contracts with our significant others. Therefore, we don't honor our contracts with ourselves. It appears that our lack of commitment to honor any obligation contributes to us failing to reach any significant goals. As we see, the goal of staying married has obviously been difficult for some. My personal belief is that it is because many of us have not internalized the definition of commitment. Based on the definition of commitment, which is a pledge or promise, you know dedication. Also, when you lack commitment, there is a great chance that you lack determination.

See, determination is to set bounds, to render a decision to reach a conclusion after study and consideration. Consequently, because we do not truly understand the true meaning of commitment or determination, I believe it is almost impossible to process the binding agreement between two or more parties who agree to do something, which basically defines the term contract. How can we expect individuals to honor their commitments, obligations, and be determined when they have not yet comprehended the definitions of the term contract?

Chapter 2

The Jezebel Spirit

You know you should never put yourself in a situation that you may be tempted to violate or contradict any of your spiritual or moral value systems. See, the devil is really tricky and comes in many forms. In fact, he can come in forms such as friends and family members, even in the form of our very own children.

Believe me, when the devil is busy at work, he attempts to deceive you in all sorts of ways. Individuals who you have not heard from in years begin to call; you start to run into your old girlfriends/boyfriends/sex partners and associates that you haven't connected with in years—they just begin to pop up everywhere.

Those ungodly spirits and thoughts start to come and attack you, and if you are not prayed up, you will succumb. That Jezebel spirit begins to take over those old associates, and they begin to attack. Again, if you are not prayed up and covered in the blood of Jesus, you have a vicious fight ahead of you. By no means at anytime one should become arrogant because when you are arrogant you are at your most vulnerable point. The reason why is because you don't feel that you have anything to worry about or prepare for; therefore, when the devil pitches a fastball and you are accustomed to the knuckleball, that's when he gets you.

As I said earlier, he comes in many different forms; therefore we have to be ready. The devil came in the form of an old associate/friend whom I hadn't seen in years. At the time, I didn't think much of it; it was very nice to see someone whom I hadn't seen in a while, so we exchanged numbers. I had no idea that the very act of exchanging numbers would significantly impact and alter the entire course of my life.

I remember our first conversation; we talked a little about life and how things had been going since we last saw each other. The last time we saw one another was years ago when she was experiencing a very bad divorce, and I remember she was very upset one day and I took her home because she was in no shape to work. It had to be three or four years or so between that time and the time that we reunited that day at the credit union. Well, the exchange of numbers led to small talks. Like I said, we were doing a little catching up.

At the time, I had been separated from my wife and had filed for a divorce. I was only waiting for the courts to advise me of the final decision. It really should not have taken as long as it did because we had a prenuptial agreement and we had possession of all of our respected properties; nevertheless, it took some time. In the meanwhile, we would talk about life and our experiences with divorce. I really felt comfortable with her because after all, I was there for her when she was going through her divorce, and I really thought that she was there for me. Maybe she was, maybe she wasn't; however, I should not have been in this situation.

Well, like the saying goes, familiarity breeds contempt, and this comfort cost me dearly. We began to hang out more and more, hanging out around the house, and getting comfortable. I remember even hanging out with her on that Thanksgiving. I also remember saying to myself, "Why am I even here, but this won't lead to anything because she's only a friend, and besides she has my back, nothing won't happen. And if anything even appears that it will happen, I will handle myself appropriately."

I have my own saying that I often reflect upon during a lecture or when I am doing a motivational speech: "Denial is a terrible disease because the one thing about the disease of denial is that you don't realize that you have it." Well, what can I say? I had some major denial issues going on at the time. My denial was so bad that I continued to say to myself, "It won't happen to me." Well, to say the least, it did.

One day I was just in a terrible funk; you know when you are just going through and your thoughts are all jacked up and you are just hurting. At the time, I was reflecting back on the good times with my wife but also saying that I didn't want to go back to the drama. But I really and truly loved this woman more so than I ever loved anyone. I was a HOT MESS! My emotions were all over the place. I don't know who said that men don't have emotions because I was all jacked-up and couldn't get my mind right at the time.

Michael Baisden was right on track when he wrote "Men Cry in the Dark," because I definitely did more than my share of crying in the dark. I remember crying so much one night that my pillows and bed looked like someone poured a half gallon of water on them. I was really missing my wife and the life that we had, but this time I just couldn't pull myself together to stay in the marriage because I know that it would be OK for a moment, but eventually it would fall apart as it always did in the past. I knew that I needed to talk to someone, but I didn't want to talk to any friends because they all knew what I had been through before, and they all were so very supportive, and I also just wanted to hear someone else's opinion.

So one evening I asked her if I could come over because I needed to talk and get her opinion on what she thought about the feelings that I was experiencing and how they compared to hers during her experience. I, being a professional, should have never been in a situation like so; however I just wanted the opinion of a person who did not have the influence of psychology or any training, just someone who I thought would just be sincere in giving me their honest thoughts. Therefore, since I did know her for approximately thirteen years, I assumed (we all know about assumptions) that it would be safe to disclose what I was feeling. As I began to talk to her, so many emotions began to surface. I cried; I got angry, frustrated, and confused.

As I said earlier, I was a HOT MESS! I can't say that during this time I was at my best emotionally, and therefore I know I wasn't thinking straight. The reason

I wasn't thinking straight was because I wasn't where I was supposed to be in my walk with Christ. What I didn't realize was this: "Without Christ, man finds himself in situations where he knows what is the right thing to do, but is unable to do it" (Romans 7:15, 18–19). So therefore, I didn't exercise the discipline to do what I knew would occur when those feelings of lust and emotions began to take over.

At this time I was only being self-centered and self-serving, and consequently I found myself in a situation that I knew I shouldn't have been in. This was so very obvious because as soon as this sinful and lustful act occurred at that exact moment, I knew that my life would be forever changed. I immediately jumped up and fell to the ground and wept, knowing that I was wrong and this should have never occurred. My mind was so cloudy, and I was so confused, frustrated, and absolutely disgusted with myself. Something within myself was telling me that "brah, you have just conceived a lust child."

For the next few days, I found myself thinking about what I had done and what was going to happen. To this very day I still think about that moment that changed my life. I couldn't shake it off; in fact I was depressed and wasn't having many positive thoughts about living. This was really devastating for me, and the Lord only knows how my parents would respond to this.

My biggest fear would possibly become a reality. Well, it did approximately two weeks later. It could have been longer; don't hold me to that time period. Nevertheless, my biggest fear did in fact become a reality. The results of the home pregnancy test were positive. At this time, major panic and denial began to set in. Another test was taken, same result. I said to her, "You're pregnant." I then became very quiet and left. Once I left, all I could remember was total numbness as I drove for hours and hours, finally stopping at a canal and having some of the most irrational thoughts.

Chapter 3

I Told You

I remember years ago when I was testing to get into law enforcement, I had to take a psychological examination, and one of the test questions was, have you ever thought about committing suicide? Well, I can't say that I thought about suicide but I really wasn't happy about living at that time. I knew suicide wasn't an option but I had a ton of emotions and irrational thoughts.

I remember thinking if I could find a way to die or get killed and not have to do it myself. I also knew that suicide was not an option because my soul would be forever damned and suicide was the only sin I could not be forgiven for. Besides, that was the easy way out, and I always prided myself on being a "MAN" and not an

"ADULT MALE," and I could in no way not "MAN UP" and fulfill my responsibilities as a man if she were to have this child.

But in the meantime, I continued to beat myself up mentally, emotionally, and morally. I felt so guilty because throughout my life, I prided myself for not ever having a child out of wedlock. Moreover, I knew that it was wrong, and I didn't want to be a statistic. Well, I became both a statistic and another brother with an illegitimate child. I was so ashamed and guilty of the prevailing situation. I don't believe a day went by that I didn't cry for hours. I said to myself over and over again, "I can't have a bastard child."

It was so hard for me to shake off these feelings and emotions that I was experiencing. I knew that I didn't have any emotional attachment to the child's mother, and it was certainly going to be a very difficult time trying to love a child of someone that I didn't love myself. I knew that I had to work through this, and the only way was to go to my Lord and Savior.

During this time of devastation, I did something that I had not done since I graduated from high school and that was sleep under my parents' roof. I was going through it and really needed the comfort of my parents. I remember being terrified about telling my parents about what I had done and feeling that the world would judge me for what I had done. I trembled as I told them that I had conceived a child with a woman who was not my wife. I held my head down in shame and told them that I wouldn't blame them if they disowned me because I really messed up.

To my surprise, they embraced and hugged me and said that it was going to be all right. At that time I felt a million times better and felt a huge burden lifted. Over the next few days we prayed, talked, and prayed some more.

My parents and I fasted for thirty days for a blessing and a breakthrough. Now the breakthrough that I had on my mind was for her not to have the child so I could move on with my life but that wasn't the Lord's plans. His plans were for me to accept the outcome and continue to serve and trust in him regardless of what the circumstance looked like.

It's funny that when we are not a part of a bad situation, we can tell others to accept things, but when the shoe is on the other foot, it becomes so difficult. However, ever since this situation became a reality, I had the serenity prayer on lock. For those who have never heard of it, it goes like so, **"Lord, grant me the serenity to accept the things I cannot change, the courage to change the things I can, and the wisdom to know the difference."**

This prayer has certainly empowered me, and I live this, not just recite it. Well, anyway, my faith would be tested because as previously stated, what I wanted was for her not to have the child, but that wasn't the case.

Allow me to digress. When we both discovered that she was pregnant, I immediately had this stunned look on my face, and if I'm not mistaken, I recalled saying to her, "Well, you don't have to worry about anything. I'll take care of the procedure because you shouldn't have to pay for an abortion." Now this is not a unique response when a man is approached by a woman telling him that she is pregnant from him or he is not in love with her or even in a committed relationship with her.

This is what I don't understand about some women: when a woman tells a man that she is pregnant and the man responds with that dumb look on his face and he is not as enthusiastic as she is, then both should know that they are not on the same page. This is the beginning of some heartaches. And if you misinterpret the body language, I may try to give you guys the benefit of the doubt (not really). But how in the 'H' 'E' DOUBLE HOCKEY STICK do you misinterpret, "I'll pay for the abortion."

I believe this is denial exemplified through what I call the RRJ process. This is when individuals romanticize relationships that they want so bad. Rationalize regardless of the circumstances or conditions. And justify when it does not turn out the way they wanted it to. I'll stop there with the RRJ process; you will get more on that in the very near future.

Nevertheless, many women go on with this fantasy that he wants the child just as much as she does regardless of his actions and words. Only time and hard time forces women to understand that his actions and words were consistent with each other. The unfortunate thing is that a woman's denial can lead to resentment for men, which normally sabotages their future relationships with other men.

Also, another side of this crazy situation is that many women fail to realize that this is just the beginning of a crazy cycle of threats, retaliation, slander, courts, and pain. In my opinion, the pain of rejection is the most significant of this entire ordeal. Because after all, who wants to be rejected? However, I believe that there is more to just the personal rejection that women deal with; there is also the rejection of the child that she is now carrying. I can't even begin to imagine the amount of pain, however, because I am writing this book and have interviewed countless women, it's quite obvious that the pain is quite severe. The pain doesn't just last for the nine months that she is carrying but possibly a lifetime of counseling, support systems, forgiveness and prayer. This can be very challenging especially when the other party is being extremely difficult and asinine and refuses to be a part of the pregnancy and refuses to take responsibility for their part. What I am about to say will be very difficult for the reader to digest, but it is very necessary. In fact, it will stir up many emotions, but hopefully these emotions may help those who read this book solve many of their problems before they occur again.

I want each person that reads this book to think back and attempt to remember if he or she has ever heard of the term "deadbeat dad" or the phrase "how can he/you make a child but don't want to take care of it?" or "I'm good enough to lay up with, but I'm not good enough to have your baby." These are just a few statements that we often hear from or say to the other party involved.

Nevertheless, I want every woman reading this text to pay very close attention to what I am about to say. Please, please process this and think very hard on it. First, I would like to ask you, would you invest or sacrifice your time and money to Terri Rahrah? Who is Terri Rahrah? Terri Rahrah represents a perfect stranger or someone who a person is emotionally disconnected with party involved.

I am giving this example of Terri Rahrah to help those who may have said to the child's father, "You're a deadbeat. How can you have a child and act as though you don't care about it?" See, the fact of the matter is that he does not love you nor was a child part of the scenario. Unfortunately, your poor judgment of character and your bad decision to lay up with someone who does not care or even loves you has you asking these very questions.

Most males aren't willing to sacrifice their time, money, and emotions into anything that they do not care about, so if there are any limitations on any of these, then you can just forget about it. There are exceptions to the rule; however, this is the norm. My personal experience was that I was extremely irresponsible and the one that I brought into this world I had to take care of.

The little one did not ask to be here, and I have a great responsibility to provide, care for, and nurture him. Now, before you get all teary-eyed remember I had some serious emotional struggles about his existence. I knew that I had an obligation to take care of him, but loving him was something that I really and truly struggled with. For years I couldn't say that I honestly loved him like I did my eldest.

I did everything not to display any signs of not loving him; therefore at times I overcompensated with making sure that he had everything and anything thing that he needed. Nevertheless, that genuine, internal, natural, and innate love for him did not exist. It's not right, but it is the truth, my truth, and I believe that this is many others' truth, but I am strong enough to acknowledge my struggles.

So in order not to get myself in trouble with my Lord and personal Savior, I had to do right about him. So not only did I repent from this very sinful act that I committed, I refused to compound this situation with being irresponsible and not taking care of him and abandoning him. I believe that when we neglect to take care of our responsibilities, there are serious spiritual and social consequences. Here is something that I have to say about what happens when we continue these patterns, and it's called **"We Have Lost Our Position."**

Yes, I truly believe that we have lost our position within the household, the church, and in society. Our women have become the backbone of society as they are in our household as well as in our churches. It has been increasingly common to see the home headed by women. Also, the same applies in our churches especially when you consider the female membership compared to male membership. It's quite obvious that we need to reclaim our position. But first we must reestablish our relationship with God so that he can give us the guidance and ability to stand fast, so that we stand and hold the position that he had us to be in.

We must follow his direction and abide by His commandments. This is the only way that we as men can reclaim our position within our society. We have become so complacent with not having the responsibility of taking care of our families and our children but placing the burden of responsibility of taking care of our children and placing it on our women; we have lost our favor with God. Men are here to lead nations, to take care of their families, to provide for them, and to lead and guide their families in the word of God. Unfortunately, we're not doing so and caring for our families and doing the will of God. We are not taking care of our children. We are not taking care and leading our wives like we should. We continue to fail our families, ultimately failing God. According to 1 Timothy 5:8, "But if any provide not for his own and especially for those of his own house, he has denied the faith and is worse than an infidel."

These are some strong words in this particular verse; however, it's reflective of our world and what I see in our society today. Men today must realize that their blessings will continue to come short because we continue these patterns. Our actions are not in God's favor. He did not put us here to abandon our offsprings and wives (women). We have a responsibility to lead, love, nurture, and take care of those within our household. How can we say we love God and don't love our families? It's easy to say, "I love my kids, I love my wife," but the way we leave and abandon them is not reflective of love. It's reflective of being an infidel. It's reflective of denying the faith and denying the will of God. It's no wonder that the order of society has changed.

Chapter 4

The Threats

When it was discovered she was going to have the baby and I wanted to work things out with my wife, the phone calls began. The phone calls were relentless with demands. Although she said she was fine with my decision about our situation, it was evident she only said that to save face and was not being completely honest. She obviously was hurt and felt alone, but believe me, having this child was not something I wanted, and I wished it all could go away.

Nevertheless, that was not the case; we both had to deal with the reality that our lives were going to be significantly altered. So we were off to the races of emotional turmoil. According to the Webster's pocket dictionary, turmoil is defined as "a disturbance." With that said, my life as I knew it was going to be majorly disturbed, and her phone calls were the weapon of choice she used to begin the disturbance.

At first, the calls didn't bother me. I believed that they were innocent, but after getting them a bit too regularly, I then realized that there was a motive. It seemed like I received a phone call almost every day. Each day she had some reason to give me a call and justified it each time. As time passed, her calls became more frequent and later in the night. Eventually, I found myself getting into arguments with her about issues I believed were insignificant. The redundant arguments pushed me to the point of not answering my phone when she called.

The next issue was she started demanding that I get her prenatal products and bring them over to her house. Mind you this was not a request but rather a demand. Quite frankly, it was funny to me because this woman was actually demanding that I purchase her prenatal products. She was making this demand as though I was her husband or responsible for her. What made this situation even more insane was she knew I was attempting to work things out with my wife. I truly believe she was doing everything to interfere with what I was trying to accomplish. In my opinion, she was actually pathetic; however, I was equally pathetic because I was a major part of the drama. I have to empathize with what she was experiencing.

I definitely understand she felt hurt, confused, and abandoned, and she had every right to feel this way. As for myself, there were some things I was going through emotionally. Here I was, married, I haven't interacted with my wife for approximately eighteen months, and trying to work things out with her, as well as having another woman pregnant.

In addition, I was ashamed, embarrassed, unhappy, frustrated, and overall, A HOT MESS. For those who do not understand the term "A Hot Mess," it basically means I was in a jacked-up situation or a real bad predicament. At the time, I just could not see a way out. I just had to believe I would eventually come out of this valley I was experiencing.

And I did. God was truly testing my faith, courage, and my spirit. He knew I could get through this negative situation and the agony of crying, and then crying some more. God was able to see into the future despite my confusion and blurred vision. He knew that I would be responsible, share my story with the world, and most importantly, allow others to learn from my hardships and disobedience. He did not put more on me than I was able to bear.

I sometimes wonder why I have to go through so much in life, then I consider that God has something in store for me that is bigger than I can imagine for my life. I truly hope so since I want to be a good shepherd with what he has blessed me with because that has not always been the case. Thereby, whatever my Lord and personal Savior has me to endure, this exactly what I have to do.

After a while, the threats of the prenatal care had ceased; however, there were other threats I had to endure. Yes, you already know; if you catch my drift—I wasn't going to be able to see my child. Of course when she made this threat, I told her that I really didn't care because I didn't care for her or the child in that manner. I didn't want the child, and I wasn't emotionally attached. In addition, I wanted this all to go away; therefore, this particular threat was actually great news for me at the time. It was actually music to my ears. Again, during this time, I was lobbying for an abortion, along with dealing with my personal struggles with her having this child.

However, after really sitting down and attempting to deal with reality instead of entertaining my irrational emotions, I knew deep within she didn't mean what she was saying to me. She really wanted me to connect and love this child the same way she did. In fact, there was a bit of a circular causality going on because the more she attempted to want me to be involved, which angered and frustrated her, the more I resented and was oppositional toward the whole idea of her having this child and the more she attempted to get me to make the connection and love this child the way she did. *So to keep it simple, the more she wanted something, the more I didn't, and the more I didn't, the more she did!*

Eventually, the more she realized those threats were not effective, of course she had to be more creative. This time there were men that wanted to marry her and adopt the child—she just wanted me to give up any rights that I had. I immediately said no problem! Of course this was not the response that she anticipated because there was a sudden silence.

Nevertheless, she saved face and said good because she and this individual had discussed this and didn't want any issues. When she mentioned this to me, I knew that she was at a severe emotional state, and her emotions were getting the best of her. Emotions block your ability to be sensible, rational, and logical, and obviously she was not being sensible, rational, and logical. I knew within that she was miserable and basically desperate and really wanted to know why I was rejecting her and this child that she was carrying. And she was really struggling with this and coping with this to the best of her ability. This resulted in anger, rage, and more threats. This time, one of the threats were, "I'll put you on child support."

Now if you don't know, that those very words will get a rise out of a man either through fear or resentment but at the end of the day we will respond. My immediate response was, **"Do what you got to do!"** I told her she should do what she had to do because having this child and putting me on child support was not going to make me love either of them.

In fact, I told her that when she did that, it didn't matter because all the child was going to be to me was a payment and a bill, and I was not going to feel guilty about it. Now of course those were my emotions speaking at the time, but this was how I was feeling, and women have to realize that this may or may not happen when the threats of child support are put on the table.

Many guys will either get extremely angry and resentful or conform, and based on the many child support cases in America, I believe we have the answer to that one without doing any statistical research. In fact, I have spoken to hundreds of adult males and men. The adult males opted to avoid payment and let the other parent do whatever suited them and basically not be involved with the child. As for the men, they tended to go through whatever struggles, whether they were emotional or financial; they ultimately manned up and did what they had to do and honored their responsibility.

Some have even told me that they didn't have the resources, but they would do whatever they could to take care of their child, and sometimes these could come in the form of picking up the child from school, cutting the child's hair, or providing daycare. They would do whatever they could because they did not have the financial resources. It's funny, and I say this figuratively that when guys don't want to have anything to do with the child, we hear things like "your child needs you," or "you may not have any money, but you could at least spend time with them" or "money is not everything, he/she needs their father."

But when we are committed, dedicated, and responsible, we basically have to fight to spend time with the child, to play games, chase the mother around town just to get them for the weekend and this one here: be subpoenaed to court when they know damn well you have been holding it down. It's just crazy how it is for those dealing with such issues when lust children are created. I guess that's what we get when we do things out of order.

Chapter 5

Forgiveness

Although I was going through what I perceived as hell, I really had to put things in perspective and realize and truly believe that God would see me through this and make everything turn out for the good. As I mentioned in previous chapters, I knew that I would be strong enough to get through this and responsible enough to tell the story.

During this entire ordeal, I did not exemplify strong Christian values nor did I display principles of the character of a Christian. What I did was give the image of an unbeliever. I allowed flesh to take over because I knew what I was doing was wrong but I did it anyway. Without Christ, I found myself in this situation and in a place that

I did not want to be. Romans 7 references this, so I invite you to read it.

Nevertheless, I had to get past this and step it up because the reality is I am a Christian; I had just fallen down, but I was determined to get up to address other struggles that I was experiencing. This time it was forgiveness. This was a place that I don't ever believe I think I had been before.

The teachings that I received from my parents were instilled in me. I was taught to always forgive and that God is forever showing grace to us, so therefore we have to do the same. Also, I always had this belief that there was no one worth compromising my soul for; therefore, I had to always forgive them. However, the person that I had to forgive was myself. Yes! Myself.

I needed to do something because I knew that forgiveness was not an option and it is a distinguishing mark of Christian character, and I had to do something fast. In Ephesians, Paul emphasized the true meaning of forgiveness: "Let all bitterness, and wrath, and anger, and clamor, and evil speaking, be put away from you, with all malice: and be ye kind one to another, tender hearted, forgiving one another, even as "God for Christ's sake hath forgiven you" (Ephesians 4:31–32).

During this time, the dominant image of who I was, was being challenged. For the most part I was a successful person in many areas of my life, but now I had failed to do the right things. I was going through a divorce, had another woman pregnant, and was just embarrassed about this situation that I had put myself in. Throughout life, I had pridefully relied on my own abilities, but God needed to show me that I had to rely on Him, so he put me in my place. So once He did that, it allowed me to concentrate on Him and make the right choices and get my thoughts together and get past my struggles with forgiving myself.

At this time, I knew that I was forgiven, but I had to take personal responsibility for my sins and get back displaying the true virtues of a strong believer. The English word virtue comes from the Latin word for strength, virtus. The person I am and came to be is a strong man of God, and it was about time that I claimed it again. I had to put aside the emotions, feelings, doubt, insecurities, fear, and issues of forgiveness and simply trust, believe, and obey. This lesson was basically a breakthrough that God needed me to understand for me to embrace the virtue of humility.

Yeah, this was something that I really needed in my life at this time. I needed to be freed from the arrogance of thinking that I could do everything for myself and by myself. I needed to become a meeker person and depend and focus more on God rather than myself.

Therefore, once I began to experience this virtue of humility, I submitted entirely to God and depended on Him to lead and guide me. I really had to understand that I was nothing without Him, and I had to become a partaker of Him in order to be saved. My humility had to be measured by my actions and my submission to God and not by the words that came out of my mouth. It had to be in my heart.

This humbleness that I got in learning through the virtue of humility helped me forgive myself. It also helped me realize that I had an issue with forgiving my child's mother. I was so upset with myself that I blocked it all out, but I really needed to truly address it or else how could I be delivered. As I say in this book, my lectures, and just in dialogues with people, "Denial is a terrible disease because the one thing about the disease of denial is that you don't realize that you have it." So obviously, I was in denial about how I was feeling about her and the issue of forgiveness.

As I reflect, I believe it stems from the feeling of being taken advantage of at my most vulnerable point in my life as I discussed in chapter 2. During this time I was going through a divorce, eighteen months had passed, and I was really missing my wife and was beginning to have second thoughts but was not quite sure what to do. HOT MESS, remember! Nevertheless, a breakthrough was very much needed so that I could get to the point where I needed to move on. Well, thank God. Many times we feel that we are the only one going through H E DOUBLE HOCKEY STICK, but the reality is that we are not. And as much as we say that we are children of God, He got our back or we don't have a thing to worry about because we got faith; but let me tell you, stress plus flesh equates to a ***carnal mind***. We start thinking crazy; we start being all irrational and try to handle things ourselves.

The funny thing is that we pray and ask God to deliver and help us through these trials, but we don't have the patience to deal with it ourselves. I believe that God sits back and watches us make things worse so that we can realize that we can't do it without Him and realize we need to be humbled by that experience.

I thank Him for his grace and mercy because it has allowed me to learn from these experiences, ultimately making me a better man, a better father, and a better Christian. "*Nay, in all these things we are more than conquerors through him that loved us*" (Romans 8:37). Had it not been for God, "***never could have made it!***" I remember when I first heard that song. I was driving on the expressway, and I began to cry uncontrollably like I am at this very moment . . . sorry but reflecting back, this is extremely emotional for me, and sometimes I am set back. But anyway, the song was so powerful because truly if it had not been for God, there was no way that you, I, or this planet could have made it.

God has blessed me with this victory to tell my story through writing this book and allowing the world to finally hear about issues of the heart from a man's perspective. So many times, our society only hears or sees the woman's viewpoint about these very emotional and sensitive issues through books, movies, documentaries, or the media, but I am so grateful to God for giving me the strength to tell people about my experience—experiences that so many men have but no one gets to hear.

Chapter 6

Hurt People Hurt People

We all heard this before, and many of us are familiar with the emotions that go along with when we are hurt or have been hurt. Sometimes we deal with the pain in a decent way, and sometimes we don't. Sometimes we go to counselors or therapists, and sometimes we don't. Sometimes we go to God in prayer, and sometimes we don't. Well, regardless of what we do, somehow the same results occur: hurt people hurt people. It is my belief that most people are really good, but when negative emotions are involved, then that person transforms into someone else.

I remember when Bruce Banner would say, "You don't want to see me when I get mad," as he transforms into the Incredible Hulk. This is how I see individuals when their negative emotions take over and get the best of them. We become irrational, violent, and dangerous especially when we don't have adequate support systems. That's why it is so important to have people in your life who can give you that much-needed support in your time of need.

I know that many people view therapy or counseling in a very linear way; however, sometimes or most times, we truly benefit from it. I also believe that one could benefit from an accountability partner or better yet, a life coach. Therapy, counseling, or life coaching would really benefit an individual when they are faced with certain life challenges. At least they will have an outlet and professional support of someone who really cares for them and their future. However, when there is no consideration for professional services, the door is wide open to act out through our emotions. After all, when people have been hurt, they have a tendency to want to hurt others whom they feel caused the hurt that so adversely affected their lives.

Chapter 7

The Courts

How ironic is this? Exactly one year since my divorce and leaving court (**again**), this time I was back in family court for child support. Here, a marriage and family therapist in family court, back-to-back years with family issues that could not be resolved. Unfortunately for me, I was hit with a brand-new thousand-dollar-a-month bill that could not come at any worst time, especially after just losing contracts with two agencies that paid the bills.

Last year, my prenuptial saved me, but not this time. I had to pay the little one his in cash, and not love, time, and nurturing. Initially, I was a little bitter, "NOT!" Let me be transparent. I was mad as 'H' 'E' DOUBLE HOCKEY STICKS! Especially when I was still dealing with the whole ordeal of having a child out of wedlock, not to mention, that the child was conceived while I was still married; regardless of how long I was separated, I WAS STILL MARRIED! Nevertheless, I had to work through this and MAN UP!

I didn't know how long it was going to take me to emotionally connect to my child as I have with my other child; however it was not an option—I was committed to loving him unconditionally. I just did not know when that connection was going to occur. The nerve of her! There was never anything that I would not do for the little one and she knew this. So why would she do this to me? I never breached our agreement that I would basically cover all his expenses. So why do I feel screwed?

I know why. It's because I am that responsible one, and it appears that when you are a responsible individual, the organizations, the system, and especially the courts punish you, not reward or praise you for fulfilling your duties and responsibilities. Instead the courts attempted to emasculate and drain me for everything I had. And the nerve of them to ask me, "Did anyone tell you that what you did for your child is child support?" I remember my attorney (who by the way knew how I would react if confronted with such a question) tried to calm me down when I told the judge who does he think he is asking me such a question and that I don't need validation or authorization by him or the system to confirm what I am doing for my child especially when I am being very emotionally and financially responsible.

It appears that the court believes that they are the moral authority over everyone. Maybe for some but not for all. There are some of us men who had real men and fathers in our lives that were there to model and demonstrate how a real father, real man, and real human being handle their business.

I, for one, will not give credit to any institution for showing me how to be a man: neither the military, college, and especially not the courts. I have been truly blessed by several real men in my life that mentored me. This takes me back to that moment when that judge had the audacity to question me, "Did anyone tell me that what you [I] did for your [my] child is child support?" It was as though I needed him to play father to me, especially after my attorney presented documents that I had saved ever since my son was born just in case this day would come.

It's so funny that so many people say "keep your receipts, so you can have proof." Well, I am here to tell you I had four years of proof; day to day, week to week, month to month, and year to year, and somehow the courts did not take any of it into consideration. If there was any time that I lost complete faith in the courts, this was it. During that exact moment, I felt as though I was back in the fifties and sixties and regardless of how much proof I provided, there was no chance of me seeing justice. I was in a losing battle, and the judge knew it the minute he looked at me as I sat down. I could see it in his eyes, pure hatred and contempt. I'm not saying anything, but . . . all I can say is he didn't have to be so aggressive initially toward me and my attorney. You just had to be there!

During the time we were in court, I began thinking about the times when the little one's mother would call me all times of day and night demanding things and questioning me as though we were in a relationship. She would actually talk as though I had to obey her. And when I would either attempt to tell her that she could not make any demands on me because we were not in anything close to a relationship, it went on deaf ears.

At this point, she was completely irrational, and only time was going to heal her hurt heart. We know that when individuals can't manage to control us with their threats, what's their next best effort? Yeah, you guessed it! The threats of child support, regardless if you are being responsible or not.

Our women know that the system is—always for the most part—going to side with them. There I was in court, reflecting back on those many days of threats that now have become a reality. I am in court for child support, being lied on, exploited, humiliated, and most of all, hurt. Not to mention, the judge who appeared to have an unwarranted vendetta against me and my attorney as though we had slain his family. This judge did everything in his power to emasculate both me and my attorney. Had I known better, I would have asked myself, "Am I a criminal?" Because the way he was behaving in family court was reminiscent of my experience working in criminal court as a law enforcement officer after the judge was tired of seeing a defendant in court for the same infraction after he had warned them that he better not see his face in his courtroom again.

My experience in court not only challenged my belief in family courts but put real questions in my mind about social engineering and the conspiracy against hardworking individuals who do the right things concerning their children. The system appears to ignore the tens of thousands of those who have not given a dime to take care of their responsibilities. It even makes me think about those men who have proven through DNA test that the children are not theirs; however, the courts still require them to remain on child support. Just something to think about!

Chapter 8

Where Do I Go From Here?

The next day I got on a plane and headed back home to Atlanta and began writing Lust Child. I started wondering how I was going to deal with providing for my son when there was no income. At the time, I had been losing clients—in fact, it wasn't a week later that I lost my contract with the state and a local agency due to both losing state and federal funds themselves. As I remember, it was December 2007 when America was affected, and if I am not mistaken, December 2007 was the beginning of the worst economic crisis since the 1930s.

So where do I go from here? 2008 was a historic year for America. We were at the verge of having our first African American president or maybe our first female president, and nevertheless, it was a special year in American history and politics. However, it was a first for me as well. It was the first in my life that I didn't know where my next dollar was going to come from. I was struggling financially, I had lost my contracts that allowed me to support my family, and my business was hurting bad.

Basically all my life-coaching clients had stopped coming because many of them had lost their jobs and others needed to cut back on appointments for whatever reasons. I was nine months behind with my mortgage and in the process of losing my house. I was unable to find work; in fact I had applied for roughly seven hundred to one thousand jobs and positions throughout the U.S. such as Miami, Texas, Washington DC, Chicago, North Carolina, and California.

At the time, it really did not matter what city or state I was in—I just needed work. I was frustrated both professionally and personally. I needed money to keep a roof over our heads, food on the table, lights and heat on. Not to mention my obligation to the little one—he needed my support as well, and the fact that I could not provide it for him was not only embarrassing but extremely painful. I need to pause for a minute because this is very difficult for me having to write this because I was so jacked-up emotionally about not being able to really provide for the boys the way I really desire. I wasn't spending time with the little one and being a father to him like he deserved. He deserved better. Myles deserved better. Myles was with me, and he was so accustomed to having basically anything that he wanted because he worked hard for the things that he received.

This was truly a difficult time for me financially and emotionally. Times like these can make one question themselves. However, I didn't have that luxury. I knew the significance of faith, prayer, and patience. I just had to wait and see when things were going to get better. Like I put on my dedication page, "God does not put on us more than we can bear." So I had a clear understanding that I had to go through this, and I knew my Creator knew that I had the strength to bear this burden.

Of course, being the survivor that I am, I continued to seek employment, and I soon landed a position as fifth-grade teacher at a nearby elementary school here in Atlanta. The timing of this could not have come at a better time because the bank was just about to foreclose on our home. I immediately contacted the bank and advised them of my current employment, and I applied for a home modification, and I am glad to say I received one. My employment as a fifth-grade teacher was a temporary position until the school year ended. However, it was through God's grace and my faith that my Creator would provide for me and my family, blessing me to get small contracts and work here and there to keep the bills paid.

See, my favorite book says that faith of a mustard seed moves mountain, but it is my belief that doubt of a mustard seed cancels blessings. See, one should have 100 percent faith and zero percent doubt because 99.9 won't do. So that being said, I truly know that life will be challenging at times, but you have to believe and have faith, but you also have to put the work in.

Chapter 9

Clinical Perspective of Hurt and Retaliation

When an individual is experiencing hurt and emotional turmoil, their first and foremost thought is, "How can I get rid of this pain?" Unlike physical pain, emotional pain takes a much longer time to heal. Sometimes individuals fail to take time to heal by focusing on the person that caused the hurt instead of exploring areas where change is needed. After hurt had been experienced, sufficient time is not spent on the healing process and putting one's emotional pieces back together. Instead, individuals frequently make the mistake of projecting their hurt on to others, especially those whom they perceived to have caused the harm. These individuals fail to realize that the longer they fail to address their own hurt inappropriately by targeting others, the longer he or she delays the healing process.

When a woman discovers that she has conceived a child and the individual with whom the child was conceived is not as accepting or excited as she is, an inextricable level of pain and rejection takes place. Regardless of the nature of the relationship the woman has with this man, whether it is platonic or a legitimate commitment, in most occasions when an unplanned pregnancy occurs, her desire is that the male is onboard and will be supportive every step of the way.

In many instances, this is not the case when a monogamous relationship is nonexistent between both parties. When an unplanned pregnancy occurs and there is no established relationship, commitment, or attachment between the male and the female, the male normally responds by distancing himself from the situation and the female. Now there is always the exception and a very small number of circumstances where a child is conceived unplanned and it turns out favorably where both parties are onboard for adhering to their responsibilities as a parent.

The pain of rejection is a hard pill to swallow. The reality is, when a woman discovers that the individual with whom she conceived a child is no longer interested in her or the unborn child, she feels rejected and deeply hurt. In some cases, the hurt intensifies when a man tries to deny his contribution to the situation by questioning whether or not he is the father of the baby. As I discussed in chapter 3, all sorts of thoughts run through a woman's mind such as, "I'm good enough to lay up with but I'm not good enough to have your baby." This is just one of many thoughts that may run through a woman's mind when she finds herself in these circumstances.

Based on these circumstances, it stirs up rage and sometimes propels the woman to seek revenge. When this takes place, the woman is no longer operating in a rational manner; instead she begins operating out of her hurt and pain as well as her feelings of rejection. This is when the process of retaliation begins. She is bitter and no longer cares who she hurts and how she hurts them because her focus is on transferring the pain she feels on to others. What she does not realize is that the more she hurts, the more she hurts others, and in turn, the more she hurts others, the more she hurts. This cycle may continue until the woman takes time to focus on her hurt and healing, and take the focus off the individual that contributed to the hurt. Although the male is in the wrong for not taking care of his responsibilities, acting irrationally as a woman is not going to change his mind about how he feels about the situation. Instead, he will only further distance himself. What the woman fails to understand is if a man is not invested in a monogamous relationship with a woman, he is less likely to stick around and becomes even more emotionally detached if the child is conceived.

Ladies, in many cases, if the man does not have a secured attachment or verbal agreement with you, what makes you think that he will have an emotional attachment to this unborn child, which was not part of the plan? Therefore, whatever plans you have created in your minds, it will not be manifested in reality. Both parties have to take ownership of their contribution to the matter, and when they do not, it is the unborn child that suffers under these circumstances.

When a child is conceived unexpectedly to a man and a woman and there is no emotional connection that exists between the two, a certain stigma is brought upon that child. Society may have us believe there is no stigma because of what has become a normality of how our children come into this world, but believe me there is, and it hurts. Just ask.

Many do not consider the social and emotional implications that a child endures when born under these circumstances. As the child matures, deep down he or she is aware that his or her birth was not planned, and with that comes unspoken rules. The child may suffer from insecure attachment issues, identity crisis, lack of security, and an overall lack of sense of belonging. Feelings of abandonment sometimes run huge among children that were born unplanned to two individuals who share no connection other than the fact that they conceived a child together.

Think of how difficult social gatherings may be or the relationship with a sibling, which can become a rivalry if other siblings exist. The lust child may be known as the outside child or unwanted child by the other siblings or other family members, one who is considered the family's secret. Tension automatically stirs up in the air when this child makes his or her presence known.

All the while, the lust child desires to be a part of a stable family and have a sense of belonging. However, the lust child is grandfathered in by relatives because it is the "right" thing to do. Although this child did not ask to be born under such circumstances, he or she experiences the brunt of family conflict that is generated from this type of union.

Another component that the child born out of lust and not love is exposed to is the tug-of-war that often takes place between parents that have no connection to each other and are out to inflict hurt. There is often conflict centered around decision making pertaining to the child. When a man who was previously uninvolved with his child decides that he wants to make up for lost time and reconnect, the mother of the child sometimes hinders the interaction due to the hurt she experienced. This may come in the form of the mother restricting any form of contact between the father and the child. Also what happens is that the mother may transfer her pain and anger toward the child's father on to the child by verbally demeaning the father in the presence of the child. While she may be open to accepting financial support from the child's father, she is rigid regarding the father developing a relationship with his child.

Children need much more than just financial contribution from their parents. They need love, stability, acceptance, trust, and mental stimulation.

What parents fail to realize is that when one parent demeans the character of the other parent in front of the child, the child feels attacked and is placed in a position to choose between either parents. No matter how ineffective a parent is, his or her character should never be devalued in front of the child. Children are very perceptive, and they can observe on their own what is really occurring and how their parents really feel about them. The constant tug-of-war impacts a child's self-esteem and his or her ability to perform to his or her full potential. Ultimately what parents need to realize when they are in this situation is in spite of their pain, hurt, and bitterness and the fact that they may despise the other parent, one has to consider what is in the best interest of the child. After all, the child did not ask to be here, and he or she is the result of the decisions made by his or her mother and father.

Chapter 10

Nine Divine Personal Responsibility Characteristics

1. **Self-love**—One should have unconditional love for one's self because life is too precious and too short for any justification or excuses. By loving yourself you learn the significance of respecting yourself and not compromising any of your spiritual and moral value systems.

2. **Study**—Read spiritual, cultural, educational, and relational literature that serve as a support system to your personal goals in life.

3. **Have a support system**—Utilize local resources, friends, family members, church, support groups, psychotherapist, counselors, life coaches, or

organizations that will be supportive to you in your time of need. I even recommend inspirational and motivational CDs and DVDs if you like.

4. **Have an accountability partner**—These people will not always agree with you, so don't expect them to. They will not agree with you on every view, idea, or perspective, but they will be the objective that you will need at that very critical point that may prevent you from doing something that you may regret later. Like I always say, one of the most painful experiences is the pain of regret.

5. **Don't second guess yourself**—So often, we say "Man, something told me to . . ." or "something told me not to . . ." I believe that our blessings and success comes when we honor the gift of discernment. For when we go with our first instincts, excluding emotions (they can get you in BIG trouble), we pretty much have positive results.

6. **Avoid putting yourself in vulnerable situations**—As I mentioned about having regrets, placing yourself in compromising positions results in life-altering situations and may affect you financially, emotionally, spiritually, and may even cost you your life.

7. **Read positive affirmations**—Read short positive affirmations that are very powerful and inspirational for everyday life.

8. **Read proverbs**—This is from my favorite book because it is the book of wisdom and understanding. As you read it, you will learn so much about the benefits of good decision making and following the advice of the wise. Many may say that experience is the best teacher; however, in my opinion, the best teaching is by listening to the wise.

9. **Display character**—Have a distinctive quality about yourself; have moral and ethical strength. I know that we all fall short of perfection; however, I believe that we can put a little more effort in our stride to improve in the small areas in our lives. Sometimes a little more effort can lead to maximum results. And besides, what would your Creator do? Hint, hint. Character!

A Revolutionary Message

My primary objective for writing this book is for no other reason than to address or confront that "PINK ELEPHANT" that society at large which includes our educational system, our families, the church, or any organized religious institutions that refuses to address the subject matter that is in the book. This book will be like a flu shot. It hurts and is very painful; however, it is for your best interest. And like the story, it needs to be told. For anyone that is offended with this message and story, I truly apologize. It is not my intention to offend but rather to send a message of accountability and when we don't hold ourselves to a high level of morality how it affects the lives our children and the message it sends about morality and value systems.

www.ingramcontent.com/pod-product-compliance
Lightning Source LLC
Chambersburg PA
CBHW020351290526
45785CB00005B/2237